The Foot

For Healthy Beautiful Feet

Get beautiful feet with your electronic callus remover and DIY foot treatments

14 Peaks

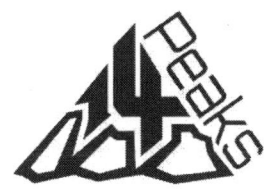

Copyright © 2016 14 PEAKS

The Foot Book

All rights reserved.

Published by 14 Peaks

Edited and formatted by La Beauté Pure

ISBN-13: 978-1544185682

ISBN-10: 1544185685

This book is licensed for your personal enjoyment only. This book may not be re-sold or given away to other people. If you would like to share this book with another person, please purchase an additional copy for each person. If you're reading this book and did not purchase it, or it was not purchased for your use only, then please return it and purchase your own copy. Thank you for respecting the hard work of the authors.

DISCLAIMER

All articles, information, and resources published in this eBook are based on the individual author's opinions and are meant only to motivate readers to make their own nutrition and health decisions after consulting with their health care provider.

Authors are not and do not wish to portray to be doctors or medical professionals. All readers should consult a doctor before making any health changes, especially any changes related to a specific diagnosis or condition. All information contained in this eBook is the sole opinion of the author and contributors.

Any statements or claims about the possible health benefits conferred by any foods or supplements within this eBook have not been evaluated by the Food and Drug Administration and are not intended to diagnose, treat, cure, or prevent any disease.

Chapter 1 HAPPY FEET = HEALTHY FEET

BEAUTIFUL FEET

A WALK THROUGH HISTORY

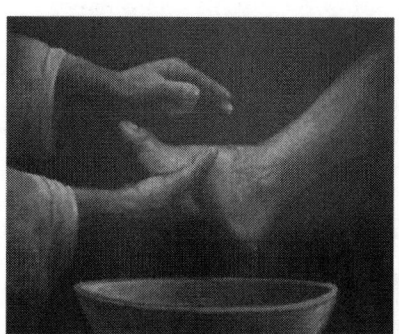

Feet have been mentioned throughout the ages in manuscripts, plays, and even in the Bible. The washing of feet was customary in Biblical days.

Men often traveled great distances barefooted or with open sandals. The host of the house would provide the water and the basin. The guest would wash his feet, or in wealthier households, a servant would do the washing. It was a sign of great love for a man to wash another's feet. Foot washing was performed for hygiene, affection, and was sometimes done ceremonially as well.

MODERN FEET: A STEP IN TIME

These days, feet are not only for getting you around, they are a fashion statement. Open toe high-heels show off the feet as do strappy sandals and even comfy fashion flip-flops. An ongoing-trend that continues to get more and more popular each year is getting married barefoot. Foot jewelry is even stylish, like fancy ankle bracelets and toe rings.

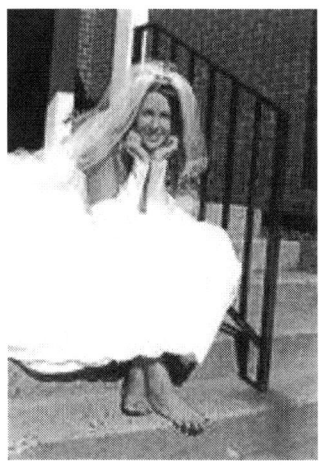 The problem is that we spend our lives on our feet, and it shows. Feet get rough, dry, callused, and just plain ugly. They are embarrassing, too! Most of us try to hide our rough, callused feet. We can pull this off for a little while, but then there comes that time you simply have to take your shoes off!

We, the people with callused feet, know that sinking feeling when we are asked to remove our shoes at the front door or take them off at a Japanese restaurant.

And…what about your favorite pair of flip-flops or that awesome pair of new sandals you have tucked away in the closet? Besides, we all love going to the beach, and it's really hard to hide your feet at the beach!

The fact is…life can be hard on your feet! You can now sluff it off with a foot care regimen including a callus remover and DIY foot treatments. Millions of dollars are spent on pedicures yearly by both men and women. Now, you can save tons of time and money by performing your own pedicure with electronic callus removers in the privacy and convenience of your own home. And…no appointment is necessary!

You can get an electric callus remover on amazon or at any drug store. The roller head buffs hard skin off instantly. In minutes, your rough dry feet will be smooth and silky.

Well, most feet. This is for average feet. If you have built up thick hard calluses, it may take you several sessions to get silky feet. You can certainly do it all in one session; it just takes a little longer.

HOW DOES AN ELECTRONIC CALLUS REMOVER WORK

Using the electronic callus remover is super simple!

To get rolling:

>Step 1: Wash and dry your feet.

>Step 2: Lightly move the unit over the callused area until the dry hard area is smooth.

>Step 3: Cleanse and moisturize your feet.

>Step 4: Go show off your new silky, smooth, beautiful feet!

It is recommended that you exfoliate your feet once a week. This can help you avoid having to spend a long time in one sitting.

WHY USE ELECTRONIC CALLUS REMOVERS?

It is estimated that 87% of adults in the United States alone have some type of foot problem. One of the most common problems is calluses.

What are calluses anyway? Calluses are thick and rough dry patches on the skin, commonly occurring on the bottom of the feet. They are usually caused by repeated friction, like walking a lot or wearing shoes that rub. As we age, calluses form over the years, even on feet that have been well taken care of. Calluses are just an inevitable fact of life that many of us have had to endure.

Calluses can be painful, especially if the hard, dead tissue fills up pores and sweat glands. Calluses can become infected. They can become ulcerated too. Athlete's foot is another condition that goes hand-in-hand with callused feet. When your feet are in poor condition, it causes stress, giving you unhealthy feet.

In addition, calluses can affect your posture, causing chiropractic issues. It is imperative to take good care of your feet. After all, they are the only ones you will ever get. They have to last a lifetime.

Exfoliating the affected areas with a callus remover will smooth and soften the rough hard calluses right off. If your dry rough feet have not escalated to the point of being callused yet, they don't have to. You can stop the process now. With regular use, you can prevent calluses from ever occurring.

Don't let good feet go bad. If you are one of the fortunate ones and your feet are practically perfect, electronic callus removers will help to keep them that way.

THE MAN, THE MYTH, THE MACHINE

It's a complete misconception that taking care of your feet is feminine. Tending to rough, dry ugly feet is anything but gender specific. Men often have jobs that require being on their feet or they participate in sports, like soccer and football, that can cause their feet to suffer.

Not only do these manly activities tend to cause callused feet, callused feet also tend to interfere with doing those activities. It is an endless circle that can be stopped. Besides, everyone deserves to have healthy, good-looking feet. Real men DO use callus removers!

FOOT FACTS:

- The average person will walk over 100,000 miles in a lifetime. That's like going around the entire globe four times!

- Just wearing a 2½-inch high heel can increase the load on the front of the foot by 75%.

- Women are four more times likely to have feet problems. This is oftentimes due to shoes with the priority of fashion over comfort.

- In one day of average walking, the forces impacting your feet can total hundreds of tons. That's the weight of a fully-loaded cement truck.

- Your feet have a lot to do with what happens in other parts of your body too. On each foot, there are over 7,000 nerve endings called reflexes that correspond to every organ and system in the body. By pressing on the reflex point, you stimulate the nervous system and open energy pathways that may be blocked or congested.

- Foot conditions can become your first sign of a more serious medical problem. Your feet are the mirror of your general health. Arthritis, diabetes, nerve and circulatory disorders, as well as other conditions, can show their first symptoms in your feet.

- There are 3 million sweat glands in the dermis of the adult foot. Feet need to breathe to operate properly. Clogged pores prevent this from happening.

- We all enjoy a good pedicure, but did you know that bacteria and fungus can easily move from one person to the next in a salon if they don't use proper sterilization techniques. Any cuts or open wounds are prey for bacteria. Doing your own pedicure in sanitized conditions in your own home is a safe way to go.

- Feet are the fastest area of the body to absorb things because of the large pores. While that can be a bad thing, for instance, if you are exposed to toxins via your feet, it can be a good thing too. Essential oils can be massaged into your feet, benefitting the health of your feet and your entire body as well.

DIGGING A LITTLE DEEPER: MORE FACTS ABOUT CALLUSES

- Calluses are not contagious but may become painful if they get too thick.

- The callused area is hard and shiny and usually greyish-white in color.

- In people with diabetes or bad circulation, calluses can lead to more serious problems.

- If left unattended, corns and calluses may require surgery to remove them.

- Ugly callused and rough feet keep many people from doing things they would like to do such as going barefoot on the beach, getting married barefooted or even wearing sandals and flip-flops.

ENHANCE YOUR FEET

You can maximize your spa-like experience with even more steps. One way is to indulge in a good foot soak after you exfoliate with the device.

It's a great time to rub on essential oils too, because all the dead dry skin will be gone and the healing benefits of the oils can soak right in. After every use, it's a great idea to use a high-quality foot balm.

HARMFUL PRODUCTS?

In a noble attempt to try to defend problematic feet, many do more harm than good.

Many foot products, like the skin care line, have harmful ingredients in them. Triclosan is one such popular ingredient commonly used in foot powders and foot sprays. It has been linked to heart failure, hormone disruption, and a slew of other maladies.

Petroleum products, alcohol, paraffin, and parabens are a few of the other culprits lurking in foot care products that can cause way more problems than you bargained for. It is always best to go organic, and when possible, it is even better to make your own products.

"HEELING" AND HEALTHY: BEST INGREDIENTS FOR FEET

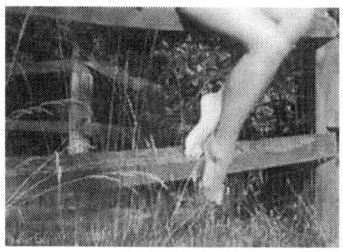

In this book, you will find some fabulous DIY recipes for taking great care of your feet, like homemade foot soaks, scrubs, moisturizers, and powders. Before we get started, here's a look at some of the very best ingredients for healthy, happy feet.

You probably have many of these ingredients in your kitchen right now. If at all possible, try to use organic varieties because you do not want to be soaking up any toxins.

GETTING A FOOT-HOLD ON NATURAL INGREDIENTS YOU PROBABLY ALREADY HAVE

Some of the best solutions for foot care can be found right in our own home. Check out these common household items and what they can do for the health of your feet.

Epsom Salts: Epsom salts are great for feet soaks, scrubs, and rubs. Epsom salt is rich in magnesium sulfate heptahydrate, which is a therapeutic mineral. It is great for muscle pain and stiffness, healing injuries, relieving stress, and arthritis, too. Using Epsom salt on your feet can detoxify the whole body.

Apple Cider Vinegar: Apple cider vinegar is awesome for pain relief, treatment of skin conditions, detoxing, pumping up immunity, controlling athlete's foot and other fungus-based conditions. It's worth noting that apple cider vinegar is best when purchased in organic form with the "mother" in it.

Baking Soda: Baking soda, or sodium bicarbonate, is one of the cheapest yet effective solutions for foot care. It can be sprinkled in shoes or directly on the feet to control odor. It cleanses, gets rid of bacteria, soothes, invigorates, and heals sores and insect bites.

Lemons: Lemons are high in vitamin C, which is rich in antioxidants. They fight the effects of free radical damage. Lemons help the feet to heal, can fade dark spots, neutralize odors and moisturize. Plus, lemons smell fabulous!

Oranges: Oranges are like lemons, extremely rich in antioxidants helping the feet to heal, controlling oils and softening the skin, and they have many terrific therapeutic benefits. They smell great and wake up the senses in addition to aiding ailing feet.

Avocado: Avocadoes are awesome for feet! They are packed full of vitamins and antioxidants, too. They heal a multitude of problems, like cracked feet, and they soften the skin.

Coconut Oil: Cold-pressed organic coconut oil is great for foot fungus. Coconut oil contains vitamin E, which is an antioxidant. It conditions the skin and moisturizes, and it is an anti-viral as well.

Olive Oil: Olive oil soothes and heals dry, cracked feet. It contains omega-3 and omega-6 fatty acids; therefore, it does a multitude of favors for your feet and can help them look younger and silkier.

Whole Raw Milk: Milk is fantastic to soften your feet and make them silky smooth. It is very soothing and relaxing, too.

Honey: Raw honey is extremely healing, and it is an oil balancer and moisturizer, too. It is a natural way to fight bacteria. Raw honey heals scars and brightens dull skin.

Oatmeal: Oatmeal in its raw, whole grain, organic form is excellent for cleansing because it contains natural cleansers called sappoins. It is also a great exfoliant, protects against toxins and UV rays, and softens dry, rough skin. It is fantastic to heal and soothe irritated skin.

SPICING IT UP WITH INGREDIENTS FROM THE GARDEN

There are spices, herbs, and flowers that can make your foot care experience simply marvelous. Mint is refreshing and soothing. Rosemary is a potent anti-inflammatory and anti-bacterial and improves circulation.

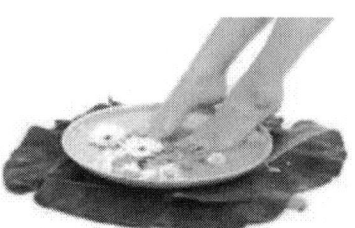

Basil is an anti-bacterial, anti-inflammatory, antioxidant, anti-viral, disinfectant, and it stimulates the foot nerves. Mint is refreshing, has a wonderful invigorating scent and is very good for aching feet. It's also easy to grow. Grab a small handful to add to the mix when blending a foot detox or soak.

Don't forget to smell the roses! Roses are healing and relaxing, too, so why not sprinkle rose petals in your foot soak or crush them in your favorite foot scrub?

SOLE SURVIVORS: ESSENTIAL OILS

Essential oils are one of the best ways to remedy foot problems and pamper them as well. Essential oils are concentrated oils, volatile and liquid aromatic compounds that are derived from natural sources, usually plants.

They are used for healing and for pleasure and well appreciated for their relaxing or invigorating effects and for their good scents.

Essential Oils come in different strengths and qualities, which makes a difference in how they will work or if they will even work. Make sure you purchase a great quality product so you aren't wasting your time and money.

Usually a carrier is required to effectively deliver the oil into your body in a beneficial way. For instance, some oils are so potent, they cannot be used full strength or they will irritate the skin or burn it. Carriers dilute the strength and help get the oil to absorb into the pores.

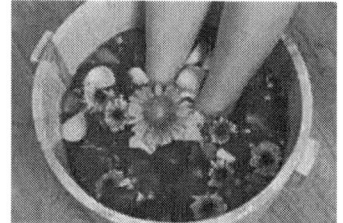

Usually a thick carrier is used for salves while medium carriers are more conducive for massage oils and thin ones are best for perfume effects or light moisturizing. Calendula oil, coconut oil, and even olive oil are great carriers that not only help transport the essential oil, but add their own benefits to the mix, too.

Which essential oil to choose depends upon which fragrance or fragrances you like best as well as the therapeutic values they possess. You can mix them into wonderful blends or use them all alone.

Here are some fabulous foot care essential oils and the qualities they bring to the table, or rather to the feet:

Peppermint: Peppermint wakes up tired feet and takes the aches away, too. Peppermint heals a multitude of ailments like pain, sores, and insect bites.

Tea Tree: Tea tree oil is like a first aid kit in a bottle. It kills germs, promotes healing, refreshes your feet, and is great for sores, boils, and insect bites.

Lavender: Ahhh...lavender smells so heavenly; it's a personal favorite. Lavender oil will relax your feet in no time and your whole body for that matter. It is also a natural pain reliever for sore achy muscles and joints.

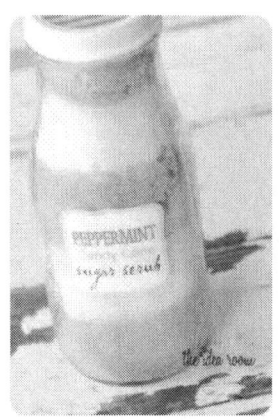

Lilac: Along with the pleasant scent, lilac heals, is extremely relaxing, and is an antiseptic, too.

Wintergreen: Wintergreen is a pain reliever and fantastic for achy feet. It has a tingling, cooling effect, kills germs, and reduces swelling, too.

Lemon: Lemon rejuvenates tired feet and helps to heal and moisturize them. It is refreshing and invigorating at the same time.

Rose: Rose oil is an antiseptic, anti-viral, astringent, bacteria fighter, and even an anti-depressant. Furthermore, it has a scent that will make your feet...well, smell like roses.

There are tons of ingredients that are super for your feet, including things found right in your kitchen or bathroom, as well as essential oils that can easily be found at the local drugstore or online.

They can be combined into intoxicating elixirs to heal and pamper your feet including soaks, scrubs, rubs, and moisturizers. The best thing about these ingredients is that they are all-natural and organic. We have put together a collection of some of our favorite DIY foot care recipes. Read on to find out step-by-step instructions to make these spa solutions. You'll be footloose and fancy free in no time.

Nature...it's good for the sole!

FOOT-NOTES

When making up a batch of our DIY recipes, why not make some extra and store it for future use or for gifts?

Many can last a good length of time in an air-tight jar and even longer when placed in the refrigerator. It's convenient to have a soak, scrub, rub, or lotion already whipped up.

Another great idea is to make extra and share with your friends. It makes a nice gift, too. You can use a mason jar or any glass bottle. Just tie a ribbon around it or place a decorative label on and there you go!

It's fun and festive to make themed foot care solutions like a Peppermint Foot Scrub for Christmas and a Relaxing

Rose Soak for Valentine's Day. It's for sure the gift that keeps on giving.

Chapter 2

THE FEAT TO CLEAN FEET: FOOT SOAPS AND CLEANSERS

Soaps often defeat the purpose of cleansing altogether. Instead of getting rid of bad things, like dirt and bacteria, they can sink poisons right into our bodies. Soaps can be full of harsh and harmful chemicals such as parabens, paraffin, cocamidoproply betaine, laurel sulfates, and other ingredients that cause a host of physical human issues and environmental hazards. But having clean feet is the first step toward good foot health. Here are some really awesome foot soap and cleanser recipes.

Lemon Fizz Cleanser

Lemon and Baking Soda are powerful natural cleansers that will leave your feet squeaky clean and fizzy fresh. Lemon is high in antioxidants, which help to repair damaged skin and protect against further damage, too. Baking soda is a fabulous natural cleanser. This lively blend smells great and is invigorating, too.

You will need:

¼ cup of baking soda

¼ cup of lemon juice (freshly squeezed)

Directions:

Place the Baking Soda in a jar and slowly add lemon juice to make a thin paste. The mixture will begin to fizz. Apply to feet and rub in circular motions, repeating for at least 5 minutes. Rinse and dry your feet.

Soothing and Gentle Oatmeal Cleanser

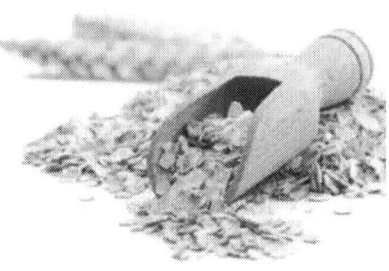

Just because a cleanser doesn't foam, doesn't mean it isn't getting the job done. In fact, quite the contrary. Soap suds are often made by harsh chemicals in a product. Here's a great cleanser that is safe and gentle for sensitive feet and highly effective as well.

Oatmeal (whole grain organic) is a miracle worker for feet issues of all sorts. It contains saponins that clean deep into the pores, exfoliates dead skin, protects the skin from harsh chemicals, and treats skin conditions like rashes and irritations. Wow! And you thought oatmeal was just a great breakfast cereal!

Yogurt (organic with live cultures and high fat content) is excellent for fighting off bacteria and is full of protein, too. It is also an awesome moisturizer and works well to soften dry patches, cracked heels, and rough feet. It contains zinc and lactic acid, so it is healthy and healing. This combination of oatmeal and yogurt is like having a world of health right at your feet.

You will need:

1 cup of organic oatmeal (uncooked)

4 tablespoons of organic yogurt (Plain)

Directions:

Mix the oatmeal and yogurt together in a jar until well blended into a paste. Smooth on to your feet and rub in a circular motion for 5 minutes with a clean, soft washcloth. You will get even better results if you leave it on for another 5 minutes, so grab a good book and relax while this awesome foot cleanser goes to work. Rinse and dry your feet.

Lovely Lavender Liquid Foot Soap

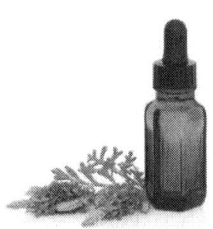

This soap is extremely healthy for your skin. Lavender has a fresh, floral scent; it is an adaptogen, meaning it de-stresses the body as it is absorbed into your feet and as you breathe it in, too.

It is an anti-bacterial and is a fantastic first aid for your feet. Now you can clean your feet in confidence and you won't believe how wonderful this soap smells!

You will need:

1 cup of distilled water

2 ounces of pure, unscented, organic liquid castile soap

¼ - ½ teaspoon of lavender essential oil

Directions:

Gently mix the ingredients together until well blended. Pour into a glass jar with a pump. Simply use on your feet as you would a regular soap. This recipe is easy to double, triple, even quadruple so it is perfect to make for really awesome gifts.

Get Pumped: Miracle Mint Soap

Peppermint is refreshing and healing. This soap will disinfect and cleanse, heal wounds, and cure aching feet. I always make a large batch so I can have plenty on hand (or...on foot, rather) to share with friends and family. It is one of my all-time favorites!

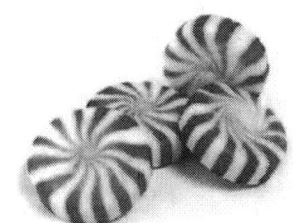

You will need:

1 bar unscented organic soap

1 gallon of distilled water

1 tsp peppermint essential oil

Large pot

Glass soap dispensers with pumps

Directions:

Pour the water into the pot and bring to a rolling boil. Shred the bar of soap into the water and stir occasionally until the soap is dissolved. Remove pot from heat and let cool, stirring every five minutes. When cooled, add peppermint essential oil and pour into containers.

From the Heart: Rose Bar Soap

This melt-and-pour soap is an easy way to make your own shaped soap from a mold. This is perfect for gifts, holidays, or just for fun. You can choose any shape and any essential oil; I love using heart molds with rose essential oils because not only does it smell wonderful, but it also detoxifies, frees the skin from bacteria and can fade scars.

Just breathing in the vapors has anti-depressant effects. The sky is the limit with this recipe. Have fun putting your personal spin on it and creating your own signature soap.

You will need:

2 cups melt-and-pour Soap (organic)

2-3 drops rose essential oil (or that of your choice)

Coloring (optional)

Heart-shaped soap mold (or that of your choice)

Directions:

To get started, cut the soap into small chunks and melt while gently stirring. Add essential oil and colorant if desired. Pour into mold and allow to sit for at least 3-4 hours. Enjoy!

Tea Tree Soap for Troubled Feet

Aside from the electronic callus remover device, this foot soap is one of the best remedies because healthy feet begin with clean feet!

Tea tree essential oil is a fantastic anti-fungal, antiseptic, and deodorizer, and is excellent to use as a first aid ointment for wounds. It heals and revitalizes even the worst feet!

You will need:

2 cups glycerin soap base

2 teaspoons tea tree essential oil

Soap mold

Directions:

Melt the soap base and blend with the tea tree essential oil. Pour into desired mold and allow to sit for 3-4 hours. Remove from mold, use regularly, and get those feet back in beautiful shape!

Chapter 3

GET YOUR SCRUBS ON...FOOT SCRUBS AND RUBS

Sometimes it's not enough to clean your feet. You have to give them a good scrub. Scrubs are designed to clean and exfoliate to get rid of rough, dry skin. Scrubs and rubs can be used in between serious callus exfoliation. Not only does a good scrub or rub make your feet look and feel soft and smooth, it is very good for the health of your feet, too. There are approximately 250,000 sweat glands in your feet. They put off as much as a half pint of moisture every day. It's not a wonder why the cells get clogged up and need to get a good scrubbing and rubbing to breathe!

"Pep in Your Step" Peppermint Rub

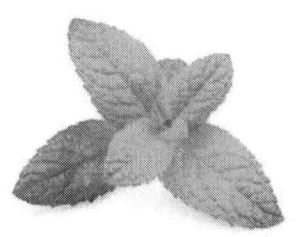

This exfoliating foot rub gets to the bottom of the problem to remove old dead, rough skin. Peppermint oil extract nourishes and heals and is a great disinfectant, anti-fungal, and improves circulation, too. It is a natural analgesic and has a refreshing tingle as it goes to work to get your feet in shape. The coconut oil in this rub is extremely moisturizing and the vinegar not only gets feet squeaky clean but heals, softens, and deodorizes. Sea salt exfoliates and contains healing qualities.

You will need:

4 tablespoons of sea salt (sun dried is best)

4 tablespoons cold-pressed coconut oil

4 teaspoons of apple cider vinegar (with the mother in it)

1 teaspoon peppermint essential oil

Directions:

Mix all the ingredients together and stir until well blended. Rub onto your feet in a circular motion using the palms of your hand. Leave on for about 20 minutes while you relax and enjoy the invigorating effects. Rinse with warm water.

Miracle Mix Foot Scrub

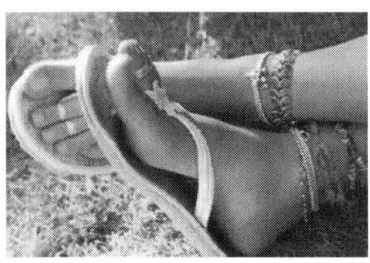

This scrub is just what the doctor ordered for weary, weathered, and germy feet. It will revive, refresh, protect, and pamper them all at the same time. And it can rid them of dangerous germs that may be lurking. I love to use this scrub after wearing flips-flips or sandals in public places like the park, the zoo, or even the beach.

It is estimated that the average flip-flop can house up to 18,000 active bacteria including the deadly Staphylococcus strain and those from fecal matter. This recipe blends the powerful anti-bacterial properties of peppermint and tea tree essential oils with the relaxing and antiseptic values of ylang ylang.

The sweet almond oil is a fantastic moisturizer for even the driest feet. You can flip the flop with this scrub, guaranteed to cleanse your feet and rejuvenate them at the same time.

You will need:

1 cup cornmeal

1/4 cup Epsom salt

5 drops peppermint essential oil

4 drops tea tree essential oil

1 drop ylang ylang essential oil

4 tablespoons sweet almond oil

Directions:

I have found the best way to make this scrub is to combine all the ingredients in a jar and shake them. Then, I let them sit in the refrigerator or in a cool, dark place for about a day.

When the mix is ready, take a small handful and massage it onto your feet.

Let it sit for at least 10 minutes letting your feet soak up the goodness. Rinse with warm water and wear your favorite flip-flops or sandals in confidence once again.

Morning Mocha Latte Foot Scrub

Want to wake up your tired feet? This scrub combines some of my favorites: coffee and chocolate. Believe it or not, both are awesome for your feet.

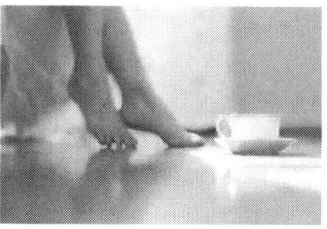

The caffeine in coffee stimulates the skin on the feet and has antioxidants as does the chocolate. The sugar exfoliates, castor oil is a natural detoxifier, and coconut oil nourishes and moisturizes. Your feet will drink in the goodness and thank you for this one.

You will need:

½ cup finely ground coffee

½ cup raw, organic sugar

2 tablespoons coconut oil

2 tablespoons castor oil

1 tablespoon raw, organic cocoa powder

Directions:

Place the dry ingredients in a bowl and mix. Then, add the liquid ingredients and mix until well blended. Transfer to an airtight jar. Scoop out a ½ cup or so and apply to your feet in circular movements for at least 10 minutes. Rinse well with warm water and enjoy your day!

Tropical Island Foot Rub

Imagine yourself on a tropical island where all your cares are cast far away. That's the relaxation you will feel with this foot pampering.

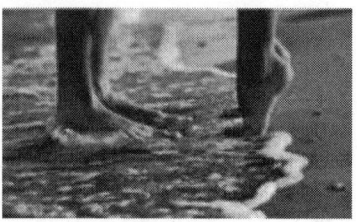

Never mind the fact that it is an anti-fungal, anti-bacterial, and antiseptic. It smells and feels too good to be concerned with all of that, or with anything else, for that matter.

This recipe uses real life white sand that is rich in granulized coral, or calcium carbonate, which regenerates skin growth and regrowth. Sea salt is healing and works alongside the white sand to exfoliate dead skin. Papaya oil is rich in vitamins A, C, and E, which are all fabulous for your skin and make it youthful-looking, too.

Monoi de Tahiti oil is made from the petals of the gardenia flower. It and the gardenia essential oil are powerful disinfectants, and the floral scent is out of this world. When life gets tough, take a walk on the smooth side with this tantalizing Tropical Island Foot Rub.

You will need:

1/8 cup Bora Bora white sand

1/8 cup sea salt (sun dried)

1/2 oz Monoi de Tahiti oil

1/2 oz papaya oil

1/4 teaspoon gardenia essential oil

Directions:

Simply mix the white sand and sea salt together in a bowl. Add in the oils. You may need to warm the Monoi de Tahiti oil slightly before adding it. Stir until well mixed. Place in a glass jar, taking out a small handful for one application. Scrub feet with circular motions, making sure to leave on for at least 10 minutes. Ahhh…it's like a vacation for your feet. Feel the difference?

Botanical Blend Foot Scrub

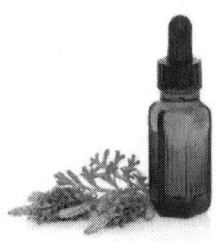

This blend of botanical essential oils and sugars will get to the bottom of your foot issues and inspire your senses as well. Brown sugar and raw sugars are both excellent exfoliates, and honey is a fantastic cleanser and healer that balances skin oils and odors, too.

Olive oil is rich in antioxidants and moisturizes tough skin. Lavender is more than just a pretty scent; it is healing and cleansing, too. The aroma of the scrub is simply heavenly and the benefits are many as well.

You will need:

½ cup of brown sugar

½ cup of raw, organic sugar

1/3 cup of virgin olive oil

2 tablespoons raw organic honey

¼ teaspoon lilac essential oil

¼ teaspoon lavender essential oil

Directions:

Blend all but the essential oils together in a bowl and then add essential oils and stir gently. Transfer to an airtight glass jar. Scoop out a ½ cup or so to massage into your feet with circular motions for 10 minutes or longer. The scent is to die for and the results are astounding. Enjoy!

Chapter 4

SOAK IT OFF: FOOT SOAKS THAT REALLY WORK

There's nothing as relaxing and healing for your feet as a good soak. In fact, it's good for your soles and your soul. Soaking your feet relieves tired, achy feet, improves circulation, softens callused areas, and even helps keep toenails clean and easy to trim. Furthermore, foot soaks are good for detoxing not only your feet, but your entire body, too.

The above is true as long as you are using the right ingredients. Many foot soaks on the market are toxic. You might actually be taking time out of your busy day to directly channel poisons into your body through your feet, so be careful to know exactly what you are soaking in and what each and every ingredient does for you…or to you.

Rest assured that the foot soak recipes here are beneficial ones. So go on, take a load off, kick off your shoes, and enjoy a nice, healthy, and very refreshing soak.

To prepare for your soak, simply fill a basin or bowl that allows a good bit of room for your feet with very warm water, as warm as you can stand it, ideally. You can place marbles or pebbles in the bottom for a massaging sensation.

Why not float some mint sprigs or flower pedals on top of the water to experience the ultimate home-spa effect? I like to turn down the lights, light some aromatic candles, and turn on soft music while soaking. No matter how you choose to do your soak, the main thing is…enjoy!

Cleansing Foot Soak

It is vital to keep your feet in tip-top condition. A whopping 75% of all Americans will experience a significant foot problem during his or her lifetime.

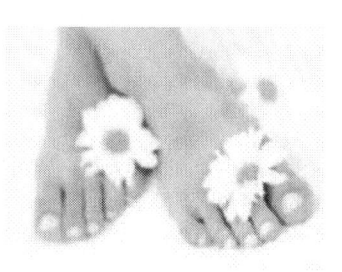

Because the average person walks up to 115,000 miles in their lifetime and 8,000 to 10,000 steps in one day, having a foot problem can be a real issue. This is one of the best foot soaks ever to ensure good health for your feet. Dead Sea salt, or even an alternative salt, helps to reduce swelling and promote healing. Lavender essential oil has an intoxicating floral aroma and also aids in the healing of wounds and sores and softens the skin. Tea tree oil has a multitude of benefits, including soothing irritations, softening corns and calluses, fighting fungus, and even eliminating ring worms.

Eucalyptus oil is like a pharmacy in a bottle. It is an analgesic, anti-bacterial, anti-catarrhal, anti-infectious, anti-inflammatory, anti-viral, and insecticidal; it is so potent, it is effective when treating shingles. Chamomile oil is a pain reliever and has many healing qualities and is very soothing to the skin. Needless to say, this foot soak is loaded with goodness and is quite relaxing and refreshing too.

You will need:

1 cup of Dead Sea salt (or sea salt or even Epsom salt)

2 drops of lavender essential oil

1-2 drops of tea tree oil

2 drops of eucalyptus oil

2 drops of chamomile oil

Directions:

Simply mix the ingredients together until well blended and store in an airtight glass jar. Pour hot water into a soaking bowl and use 1 tablespoon per soak.

Lemon-Lime Soaker

If your feet ever ache and swell, you will love this therapeutic soak. The Epsom salt aids in reducing the swelling and increases blood circulation. Lemon and lime are loaded with antioxidants that repair damaged feet and help to prevent further damage.

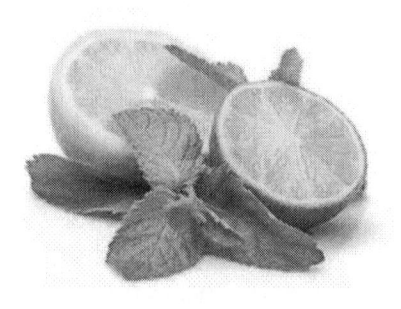

Baking soda fights bacteria and germs and is healing as well. This soak makes a really nice gift when packaged in a nice glass jar with a homemade label on it, a ribbon around it, and maybe even a little wooden scoop tied on.

You will need:

2 cups of Epsom salt

½ cup of Baking Soda

Zest of one lemon and one lime (optional)

4 drops of lemon essential oil

4 drops of lime essential oil

1-2 drops of yellow or green all-natural food coloring (optional)

Directions:

Mix the dry ingredients and then add the liquid ingredients and gently stir until smooth. Transfer the mix into a decorative glass container. Take out a ½ cup to use in your soak and store the rest in a cool, dry place.

Go Gingerly: Ginger Foot Detox Soak

This soak is such a potent detox, you really will want to go gingerly at first and build up each time you do it until you can soak for a good amount of time.

Ginger is a spice that has a multitude of holistic benefits. It is an analgesic, anti-inflammatory, antioxidant, anti-ulcer and is a very, very effective detoxification catalyst as well. So, what are you waiting for...get the lead out, literally!

You will need:

2/3 cup of Sea Salt (sun dried)

1/3 cup of baking soda

3 tablespoons of organic ground ginger

1 cup apple cider vinegar (with the mother in it)

Directions:

Combine the ingredients and place in a glass container. Start with a tablespoon of the mix in a hot soak for the first time and gradually work your way up to 3 tablespoons or even more. This solution not only detoxes your feet, but your entire body and you may feel exhausted afterward. Depending on the shape your body is in, you may even run a fever.

Don't be alarmed. It's all part of the process. Be sure to drink plenty of liquids and rest up. You will soon begin to feel terrific. Enjoy!

Herbal Essence Soaking Solution

If you are looking for an herbal experience you can sink your feet into, this recipe is for you. It is perfect for a relaxing night of pampering your feet.

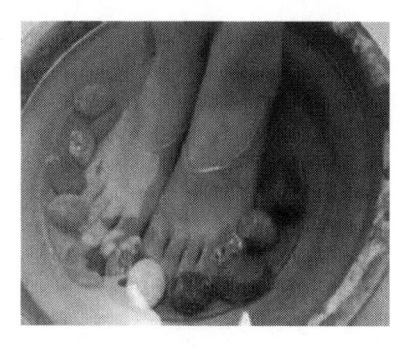

Epsom salt reduces swelling and aids in circulation while lemon essential oil is bursting with antioxidants that will revive and restore the health of your feet.

Sandalwood essential oil has a very refreshing fragrance and is an anti-inflammatory and softens the skin. Coriander essential oil cleanses and is an odor neutralizer. It fights fungus, too.

You will need:

¼ cup of Epsom salt

1 teaspoon of baking soda

2 drops of organic lemon essential oil

2 drops of sandalwood essential oil

1 ½ drops of coriander essential oil

Directions:

Mix the dry ingredients together and then add the essential oils. Transfer to a glass container. Add ¼ cup to very warm water and soak your feet for at least 20 minutes while you enjoy the relaxing herbal fragrance. Enjoy!

Milk and Honey Soak

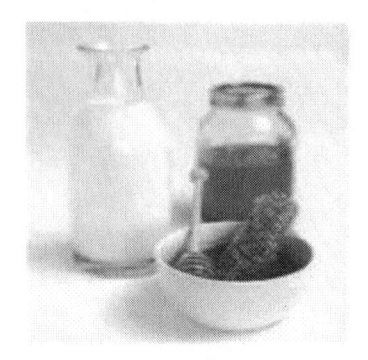

Welcome to the land of milk and honey, where health abounds and good energy flows. This detoxifying foot soak combines some very powerful ingredients that will cleanse your feet and your entire body.

It is nourishing and healing and extremely relaxing, yet invigorating at the same time. Both tea tree oil and honey possess anti-bacterial qualities and soften the skin. They are also anti-fungal. The sea salt draws out toxins and reduces swelling while increasing circulation.

Baking soda is an excellent cleanser while the almond oil moisturizes and hydrates rough, dry skin. Peppermint essential oil is healing and is a pain reliever, too. Ground ginger pulls out toxins and has many medicinal benefits. Soak it up...your feet will be happy and healthy and silky smooth.

You will need:

½ cup of sea salt (sun baked)

¼ cup of baking soda

6 drops of tea tree oil

8-10 drops of peppermint essential oil

1 tablespoon of organic ground ginger

1 cup of raw, organic honey

1 cup of organic powdered buttermilk

1 teaspoon of almond oil

Directions:

Mix the dry ingredients first and add in the liquids. Stir gently and place in a glass container. Use a heaping scoop or even two in a very warm to hot foot bath. Allow your feet to soak at least 30 minutes to reap the full benefits.

Chapter 5

FOOT BALMS AND BUTTERS, LOTIONS, AND OILS

Fancy Feet Foot Balm

This is a fabulous remedy for rough, dry feet, especially when you want to don those fancy new sandals or kick it in a pair of flip-flops. Or, maybe its winter and you know you have to take your snowy shoes and wet socks off at the door.

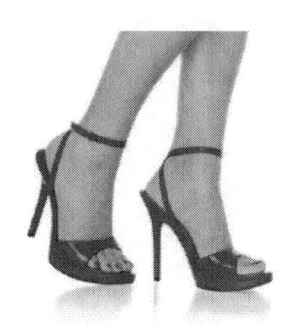

Oh, the humanity! But never fear, the Fancy Foot Balm is here. Shea butter, sunflower oil, calendula infused oil, and jojoba oil are extremely healing and moisturizing.

Tea tree essential oil is a medicine chest full of therapeutic benefits. The beeswax will seal the deal with super hydrating qualities and healing powers as well. Your feet will be silky smooth and gorgeous in no time.

You will need:

10 tablespoons of shea butter

5 tablespoons of sunflower oil

5 tablespoons of calendula infused oil

7 tablespoons of organic beeswax

5 tablespoons of jojoba oil

25-50 drops of tea tree essential oil

Directions:

Mix all ingredients together and transfer to a glass container. Apply liberally to feet, being sure to saturate the balls and heels of them where they are usually the driest. Leave on for at least 30 minutes; you can also slip a thick pair of socks over your feet and sleep with this balm on if your feet are in really bad condition. You will see the difference in no time.

Coconut Rose Foot Butter

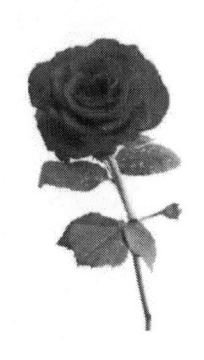

Now here's a foot solution you won't mind wearing in public. It smells really fresh and pretty, and that is exactly what it will make your feet…fresh and pretty.

The coconut oil is a healing and moisturizing ingredient as is the jojoba oil. The cornstarch will absorb odors and is very soothing while the rose essential oil is packed full of good healing qualities and smells like a botanical garden.

You will need:

10 tablespoons of organic coconut oil

10 tablespoons of jojoba oil

½ teaspoon of cornstarch

10 drops of rose essential oil

Directions:

Melt the coconut oil and jojoba oil in a double boiler and whip with a wire whisk. Remove from heat. When cooled, add the essential oil.

Heel Foot Oil

This anti-inflammatory foot remedy is also a heavy-duty anti-microbial and anti-fungal solution. It is the perfect cure for itchy, irritated, peeling, and cracked feet. Chamomile essential oil is very healing and soothing while tea tree oil moisturizes and has a multitude of healing qualities.

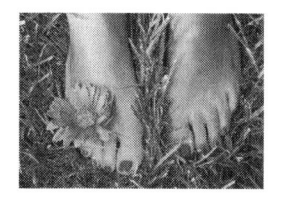

Lavender essential oil has a lovely floral scent and fights bacteria and odor, too. It is a fantastic relaxant as well.

You will need:

5 drops of chamomile essential oil

6 drops of tea tree oil

4 drops of lavender essential oil

¼ cup of virgin olive oil

Directions:

Mix the oils together and place in a glass container with a pump. Apply the intensive foot oil on your feet as needed. You can apply liberally periodically, slip socks on, and sleep in the solution. This remedy is highly effective for quick results.

Lemongrass Foot Lotion

This luxurious lotion is healing and refreshing and moisturizes even the roughest skin. Aloe vera gel is extremely effective to hydrate parched feet and to heal them as well. Beeswax is moisturizing and acts as a healing touch, too.

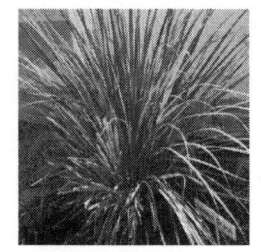

Jojoba oil has medicinal qualities and is a great moisturizer. Vitamin E is an antioxidant and moisturizer and will also make your feet look younger and smoother. You're going to love this lotion!

You will need:

1 cup pure aloe vera gel

½ cup grated beeswax (where to find beeswax)

½ cup jojoba oil

1 teaspoon vitamin E oil

15 drops lemongrass essential oil

Directions:

Combine all ingredients except for the lemongrass essential oil and heat slightly so they can be well blended. Allow to cool and add the essential oil. Store in an airtight glass container. Use as desired for a nourishing moisturizing effect.

Baby Fresh Foot Lotion

Baby's feet are so tiny and cute and soft and supple, too. You will get that baby soft look and feel with this lotion.

The coconut oil in the formula is healing and very moisturizing while the vitamin E cream is a potent antioxidant and moisturizer, too.

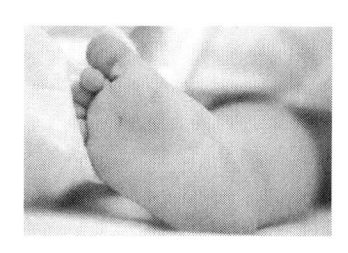

Baby lotion provides that awesome baby fresh scent and if you go organic, it will have other benefits to offer as well. Get back those baby fresh feet…and enjoy!

You will need:

16 oz of organic baby lotion

8 oz of coconut oil (cold pressed, organic)

8 oz vitamin E cream

Directions:

Simply mix the ingredients together and place in a glass jar with a pump. Use as needed or desired.

Soothing Shea Butter Bar Lotion Recipe

Shea butter is a medicinal miracle brought to you by Mother Nature herself. It is an anti-inflammatory, heavy-duty moisturizer and collagen enhancer.

It regenerates skin cells, protects against harmful UV rays, strengthens skin, stimulates superficial microcirculation, cures muscle aches, and heals minor cuts and burns.

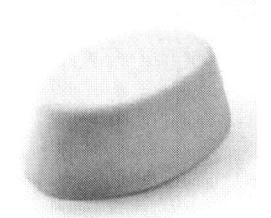

Cocoa butter is a great healer and moisturizer, too. Coconut oil heals a huge array of ailments, too. Grapefruit seed extract is one of the most overlooked remedies in existence.

It can cure many woes because of its high content of phytochemicals (types of antioxidants). Grapefruit seed extract, or GSE, is an extremely effective antioxidant, anti-inflammatory, and antimicrobial. In this recipe, you can choose the essential oil or oils of your preference according to what scent you like, what your specific need is for your feet, or both.

You will need:

¾ cup of cocoa butter

¾ cup of shea butter

¾ cup of unrefined organic coconut oil (cold pressed)

¾ cup of beeswax

1 capsule of vitamin E

6 drops of grapefruit seed extract

25-30 drops of the essential oil of your choice

Small amount of water

Soap mold, muffin tins, or ice tray

Directions:

Place the water in a medium to large pan, covering about an inch in the bottom. Place the cocoa butter, shea butter, and coconut oil in a glass measuring cup, or you can use a double boiler. Add in the wax and continue to cook at low heat until all are melted, stirring occasionally.

Remove from heat and add in essential oil and grapefruit seed extract when it begins to cool off.

When cool, pour into molds, which can be decorative ones or even ice trays or muffin tins. When they have set and dried for at least 4 hours, run cold water around the sides and bottom of the container to make it easier to pop them out.

This bar lotion is very handy to grab when your feet are in need of some TLC, and it makes a great gift to share, too!

Chapter 6

FOOT POWDERS AND SPRAYS

Sometimes, our feet have special needs. Foot powder keeps feet cool and helps absorb moisture. It's just a fact that some feet sweat more than others. Some feet stink more than others, too. Sprays and powders can help eliminate odors.

Fungal growth is common on moist feet and can cause pain and itching that can get quite miserable. Both foot powder and foot sprays can help prevent and treat Athlete's Foot fungus.

Microbial foot sprays are good to use when sharing shower areas with others such as in a dorm. Just walking barefoot or with sandals or flip-flops can expose your feet to a host of nasty things including parasites. So, get a step ahead with these powder and spray treatments.

Tea Tree Foot Powder

This is a heavy-duty foot treatment and protectant. Arrowroot powder will absorb extra moisture held around and on the feet that can lead to odors and fungal problems.

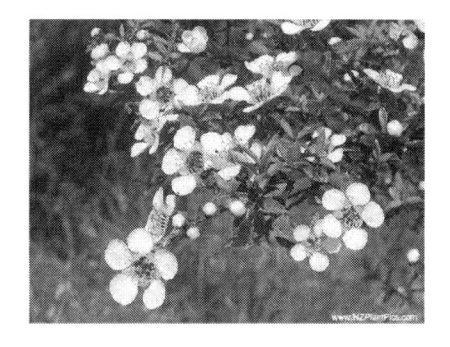

Tea tree oil is very soothing and is a very effective anti-viral and anti-fungal remedy that heals a multitude of ailments. Rosemary is healing and lends a pleasant scent to the mix.

You will need:

10 tablespoons of arrowroot powder

10 drops of rosemary essential oil

6 drops of tea tree oil

Directions:

Stir the mix until well blended and place in a glass storage container. Pinch out of container and dust onto your feet before putting on your socks and/or shoes.

Amazing Anti-Microbial Foot Spray

The lemon essential oil definitely helps to breathe a bit of life back into tired and aching feet. And the lemon juice, when it's mixed with the vodka, gives it a pretty good shelf life, too, lasting about 6 months once it's made up.

You will need:

4 teaspoons freshly squeezed lemon juice

5 tablespoons vodka

4 tablespoons distilled water

2 drops lemon essential oil

5 drops tea tree oil

1 clean spray bottle

Directions:

Place all the ingredients in the bottle and shake. Spray on your feet after entering a public showering area, after a day in flip-flops or sandals, or just for preventative measures. You can also spray this in the shower area or in your shoes or boots, too.

Minty Fresh Foot Spray

When your feet need a little pick-me-up, try this refreshing and relaxing spray-on foot remedy. The peppermint not only has an invigorating scent, but it also cures many foot ailments. It helps control foot odor and is a very effective antioxidant, too.

You will need:

1 cup of distilled water

1/4 cup of vodka

1/4 teaspoon peppermint essential oil

1/4 teaspoon of tea tree oil

1 clean spray bottle

Directions:

Place all ingredients in the bottle and shake. Apply to bare feet to protect and refresh them and to cure aches and pains as well.

Final Thoughts

Now that you know what things can damage your feet, like shoes that don't fit properly and products with chemical and toxins in them, you can concentrate on what is good for them. Regular removing of dead cells is imperative. Once you have done that, you can pamper your feet with all the wonders of the recipes you can access within this book. I hope you have enjoyed these recipes and that you now have a foothold on foot health, so yours can take you to new heights.

"A journey of a thousand miles begins with a single step." - Lau Tzu

About the Author

La Beauté Pure is all about being beautiful, simply and naturally. The business started out with four sisters, who were serious about the environment and natural products. It grew to encompass an amazing group of people, who hold the same values.

The founder, Linda, holds a degree in Naturopathic Studies and her extensive research on ingredients is priceless. She is constantly studying each ingredient in every product as well as the quality and quantity and delivery system used.

As a professional writer, Linda's sister Cheryl, took on the role of putting together the endless research that went into this book. We are all about servicing your every need and your complete satisfaction. Thanks so much for trusting us with your skin...we take that honor very seriously.

About the Publisher

14 Peaks is a publishing company that was started after the founder finished an extreme race called Primal Quest. After numerous requests for race details, the search for a platform to tell the story began. With the help of the talented CJ Jerabek, the story went to print.

After coaching for 25 years and teaching martial arts for 10, she put together a new kind of team, a publishing team. It takes a great team to help authors showcase their hard work and that is the vision. "You don't have to be an expert at everything; you just have to bring in those who are."

Wonderful, experts were brought on board that make a strong team. Professionals, who give expertise in their field, making this a winning publishing company.

Find free printable coloring pages and short stories at www.14peaks.com

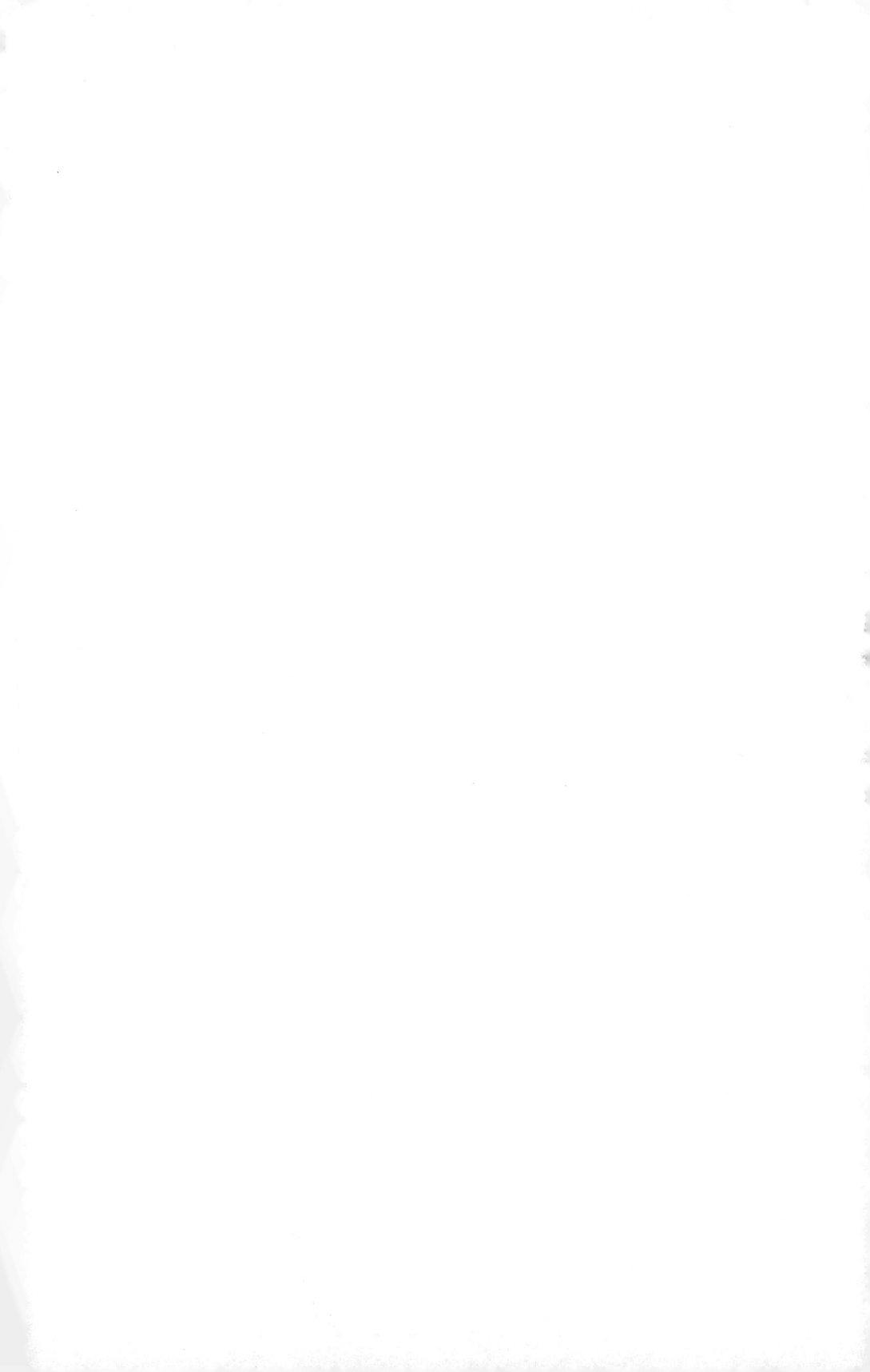

Printed in Great Britain
by Amazon